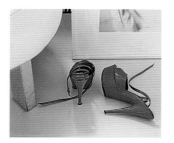

Aphrodisiacs
TOUCH · TASTE · SIGHT · SMELL · HEARING

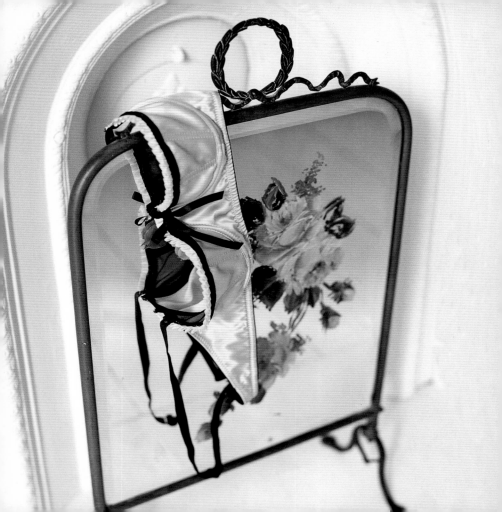

PAUL SCOTT

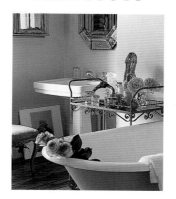

Aphrodisiacs

TOUCH · TASTE · SIGHT · SMELL · HEARING

RYLAND
PETERS
& SMALL

LONDON NEW YORK

SENIOR DESIGNER Megan Smith
SENIOR EDITOR Henrietta Heald
PICTURE RESEARCH Emily Westlake
PRODUCTION Gordana Simakovic
ART DIRECTOR Anne-Marie Bulat
PUBLISHING DIRECTOR Alison Starling

First published in the
United Kingdom in 2007
by Ryland Peters & Small
20–21 Jockey's Fields
London WC1R 4BW
www.rylandpeters.com

10 9 8 7 6 5 4 3 2 1
Text, design and photographs copyright
© Ryland Peters & Small 2007

ISBN-10: 1-84597-279-1
ISBN-13: 978-1-84597-279-0

A CIP record for this book is available
from the British Library.

Printed and bound in China.

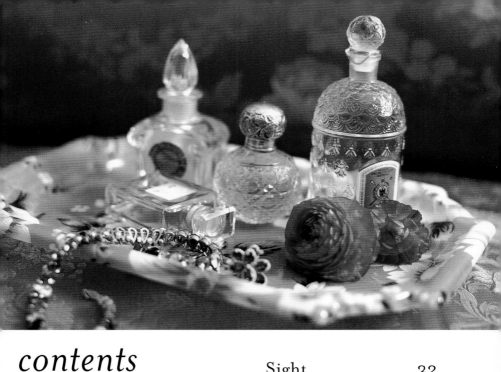

contents

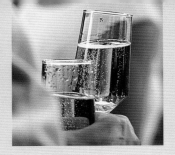

The world is your oyster

Sexual desire can be stimulated by any number of things. We are all aware of the sights and sounds that turn us on; some are ones we would expect, while others may come as rather a surprise. Our mind is the most powerful sexual organ we have, and a fertile imagination can encourage us to see sexual possibilities in even the most ordinary activities.

Genuine sexual interest such as this, together with its physical responses, is known as psychogenic arousal. This is distinct from reflex arousal, which involves only unbidden — if not always unwelcome — physical and cardiovascular changes of the kind that young men often experience as they wake up.

An aphrodisiac can be anything that has psychogenic effects, but something that is purely physical in its effect cannot be described as an aphrodisiac. Drugs such as Viagra, for example, are not aphrodisiacs. Similarly, many substances can increase sexual ability and staying power without increasing desire.

Traditional beliefs and folklore about aphrodisiacs include hoary clichés that have helped to endanger species such as rhinoceros and tiger by creating a market that has made it worthwhile to hunt these animals. The use of rhino horn and tiger penis in the preparation of aphrodisiacs is based on the theory of sympathetic magic, the belief that by consuming something you will take on some of its properties — in this case, the animals' phallic power. In an extension of this idea, oysters or figs could be said

A fertile imagination adds a sexual angle to even the most mundane activities.

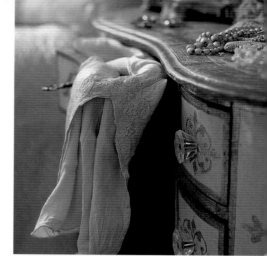

to suggest female sexual attributes, which probably accounts for their aphrodisiac associations. However, this is not to say that just because something is suggestive it won't increase your pleasure or staying power. Ginseng, for example – once known as 'manroot' – is both phallic in appearance and a genuine energy-giver.

In the short term, appealing to your partner's fantasies, spicing up your love life with sexy clothes, toys, food and, most of all, a playful attitude, will have a powerful aphrodisiac effect.

In the longer term, the most potent factor in reducing inhibitions is the trust your partner inspires in you. Your ability to listen to and empathize with others, together with a sense of humour, is the greatest aphrodisiac of all.

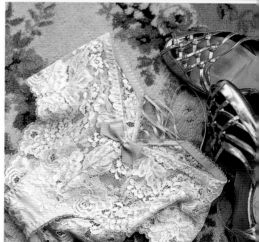

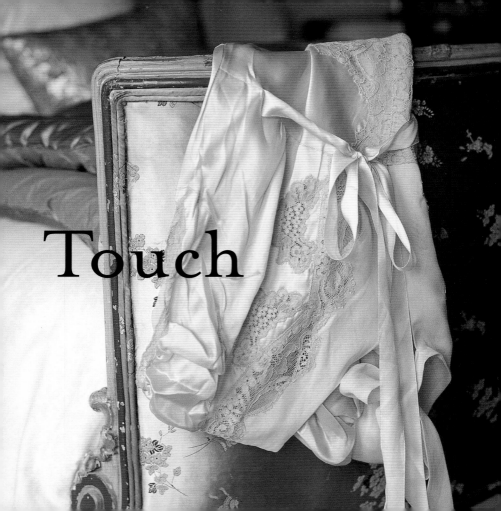

Touch

the power of touch

Our sense of touch is our most important sexual sense. While we are inclined to think of visual turn-ons when we are not actually making love, it is touch that can bring us to orgasm when we are.

Touch is the most empathetic form of human communication. To touch someone is to feel your fingers touched by that person's body, and for your lover to experience the sensation of you as if he or she had chosen to touch you, too. We touch both to explore – originally as a survival mechanism, now more often to seek out what is pleasurable – and to communicate. In the right hands, touch makes words seem unnecessary.

Experiencing sympathetic touch is a vital part of child development, and as adults we continue to need its healing power. When we are working hard or feeling stressed, it is easy to forget about our bodies altogether. Just as we get used to wearing a set of old clothes, we cease to feel the familiar, hard world around us. In contrast, we tend to remain aware of – and turned on by – the feel of well-fitting or sexy clothes against our bodies. In the same way, a simple touch can wake up our sensual selves.

With this in mind, consider the fabrics and textures you would like to fill your sexual space – cosy and comforting, or sleek, cool and sexy? It is easy to furnish a home in a way that facilitates seduction. Whatever you do, keep it warm. Poor circulation, chilly fingers and goose pimples will leave you both wanting to stay covered up!

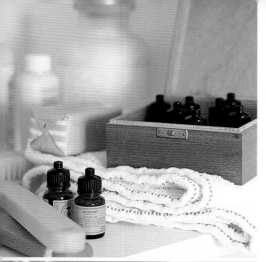

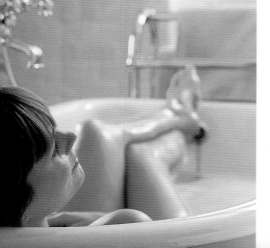

looking after number one

Feeling good in yourself will give you the confidence to have fun, to flirt and to frolic with your partner. If you are sensually generous with yourself, you will be more inclined to be sexually generous towards your lover. Giving yourself the space to compose your thoughts and look forward to the time ahead will help you to feel more in control later on.

Introducing some basic aromatherapy into your self-pampering routine is easy. Even if you've practised it before, there are always untried oils and new twists to discover (see pages 44–45).

Close any windows and doors in the bathroom. As you run warm water into the bath, add no more than 10 drops of essential oils, stirring them in so that the steam – and the scent – rises.

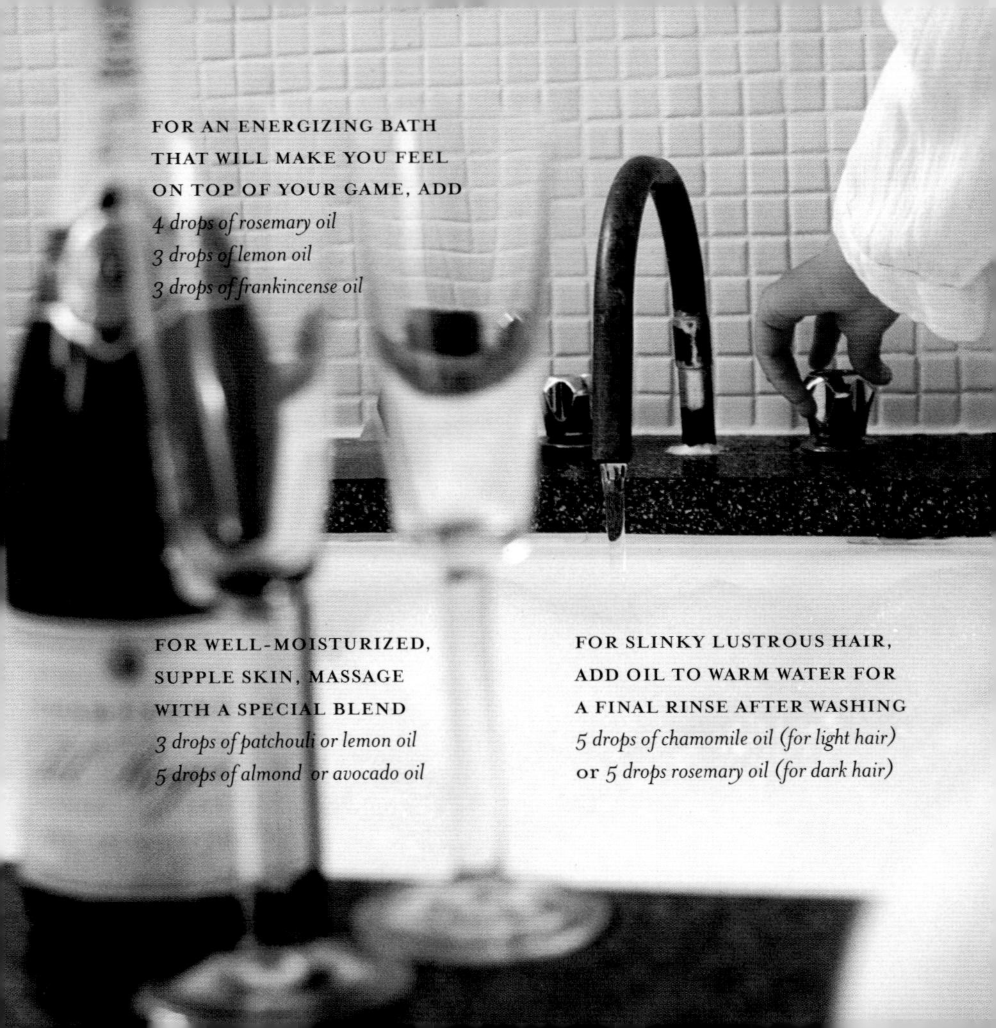

**FOR AN ENERGIZING BATH
THAT WILL MAKE YOU FEEL
ON TOP OF YOUR GAME, ADD**
4 drops of rosemary oil
3 drops of lemon oil
3 drops of frankincense oil

**FOR WELL-MOISTURIZED,
SUPPLE SKIN, MASSAGE
WITH A SPECIAL BLEND**
3 drops of patchouli or lemon oil
5 drops of almond or avocado oil

**FOR SLINKY LUSTROUS HAIR,
ADD OIL TO WARM WATER FOR
A FINAL RINSE AFTER WASHING**
5 drops of chamomile oil (for light hair)
or 5 drops rosemary oil (for dark hair)

feeling me feeling you

There are many pleasurable sensations associated with touching and being touched. If you want to enhance a sexy mood, think about how arousing such experiences can be — and remember that we feel not only with our fingers but with our whole bodies, from our temples to the tips of our toes. Listed on the right are the sources of some of the most enjoyable sensations derived from touch.

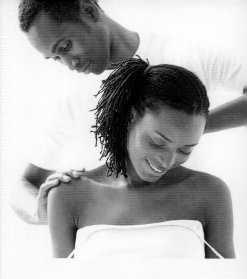

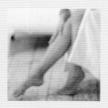

The textures of smooth and sensual foods.

The feeling of wearing clothes you know are sexy.

✳

The warmth of your lover's flushed cheeks in your palms as you kiss and make love.

✳

Fingers and fingernails drawn across your flesh — as soft and imperceptible as a hair — or waking up your flesh with a smooth, scratching action.

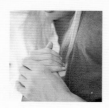

Slowly becoming aware of the gentle ache of bites and bruises you didn't know you had received because you were so turned on at the time.

✳

Kisses and tender strokes to those neglected and seldom touched areas such as your inner thighs, feet and the backs of your knees.

✳

The delicious agony of being tickled.

✳

Your lover's gloved fingers — smooth or rough in texture — in sensitive places.

✳

Little slaps that sting the giver's palm as much as their recipient's flesh.

✳

Feeling your lover's chest and groin with your back and bottom as he or she cuddles you.

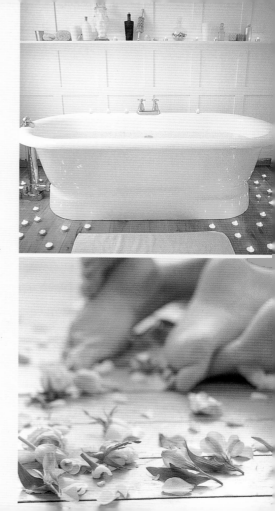

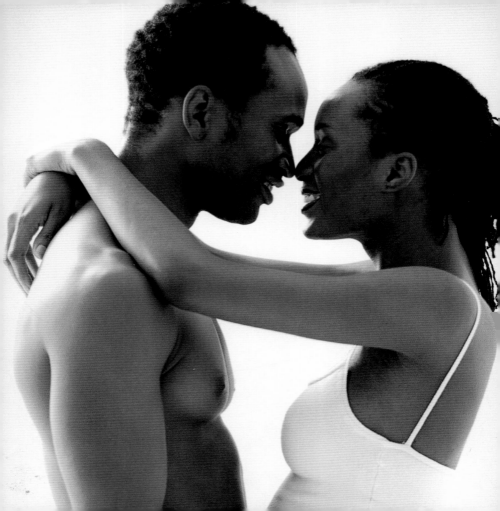

variations on a lingering kiss

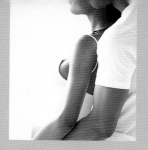

Deep, erotic kissing can be as powerful a form of intimacy as penetrative sex itself. Remember how mind-blowing a kiss can be in the earliest stages of a relationship, when you are not sure what else is going to happen and you can't take it for granted that anything will?

When we become used to thinking of kissing as foreplay, it's easy to forget the pleasure of the kiss itself. Why not keep your partner kissing for a little while? Don't be too eager to move on, treating it simply as the green light to go further. Despite their regular public appearances, your lips are made of the most sensitive skin on your whole body. Rediscover the power of the kiss for its own sake.

Grazing your lover's lips with yours can be intensely arousing. The slightest sensation, even your breath, can be felt on those rosy-red, flower-like sex organs. Whether you know it or not, the way you kiss in foreplay is a good indicator of the way you would like to go on to make love. Tender, warm and comforting — try tracing your lover's lips with a finger — or teasing and even a little spiteful.

Kissing is thought to have evolved from the passing of food from one mouth to another, and we still find it emotionally nourishing. Bestow the warmth of your lips on your lover's neck, cheeks, and ears as well as mouth. Alternatively, suck at, nibble or gently bite your lover's upper and lower lips and you'll challenge him or her to take you to a similarly borderline state between pleasure and pain.

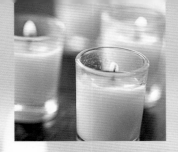

the joys of massage

When treating your partner to a sensual massage, it is essential not to expect sex. Partners who feel genuinely pampered are far more likely to respond positively. Those who feel pressurized will be tense and resentful. You are granting your lover a gift of sensations — grant, as well, the mental space to appreciate it.

A partner may need to be told to focus on appreciating his or her own sensations rather than on watching you. It is a massage not a striptease.

After removing any rings, use your fingers, thumbs and hands to feel, as much as to apply pressure; by doing this, as well as responding to loving feedback, you will discover your partner's favourite sensual treats and how most effectively to banish muscular tension.

Since your lover's body temperature will drop during the massage — more than yours will — the environment should be warm and cosy. Keep lighting low, and make sure you have enough room not just for the person being massaged but for you to move around as well. A firm surface is essential — even a sheet over a carpet is better than a saggy old mattress. Have drinks and oil to hand.

If you don't want to invest in a massage oil, baby oil or body lotion will provide sufficient lubrication. As an alternative, you may decide to experiment with essential oils blended with a carrier oil (see pages 48–49). Warm the blend between your palms before slapping it on, and remember that the hairier your lover, the more you'll need.

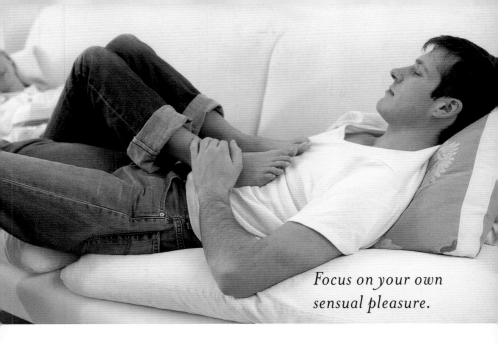

*Focus on your own
sensual pleasure.*

Keep your hands in contact with your partner's body as you massage. Begin with long strokes (effleurage) along the back, shoulders, buttocks and thighs. Kneading, squeezing and pinching muscle tissue (petrissage) breaks up fatty deposits and helps circulation. When the time seems right, roll your partner gently onto his or her back and begin on the pectorals and chest, working your way down the body to the feet, gently digging your thumbs into the soles. Experiment with genital massage if you wish. If your partner is mellow and spaced out, that's fine. But if you have opened pathways to arousal, it could be payback time.

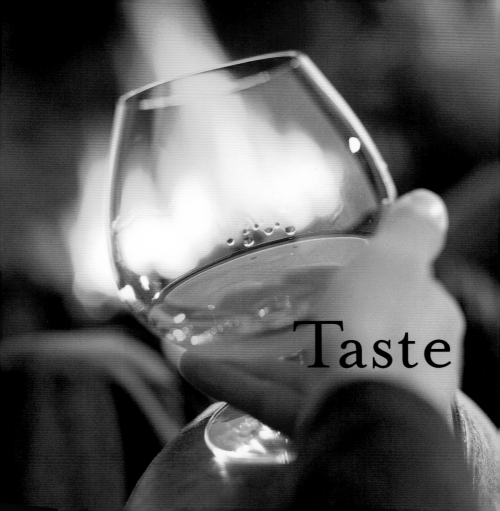

Taste

spice it up!

Food has always come before lovemaking, and not simply because going out to eat makes going home together afterwards seem more respectable. Sharing food with another person signals that you are willing to have something in common with each other, and makes it likely that the two of you will be in a similar physical and psychological state. Moreover, taste, like sex, is a world of sensation — so sharing food can be suggestive in itself.

Avoid rich foods that make you feel slothful, however tempting they may be. Fish dishes or salads will leave you nourished but not feeling as if you are bulging at the seams. This means that, if you are planning to dine at a restaurant, north Asian cuisines such as Thai or Japanese are a good choice.

The reputation of many aphrodisiac foods derives from their appearance and feel as much as from their supposed physical effects. It is not hard to see how rhino horn and tiger penis acquired their macho reputations, and the same can be said of many of our everyday and supposedly slightly naughty fish, fruit and vegetables — even if they contribute nothing whatever to psychogenic arousal (see pages 6–7) apart from their sexy shapes and succulent textures.

In the end, however, what we eat and drink in the long term has the greatest influence on our levels of arousal. A healthy diet that includes plenty of fresh vegetables and fish will benefit your overall well-being — the biggest factor influencing desire and staying power.

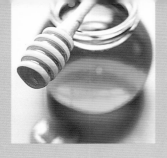

get inside your head

The value of food as an aphrodisiac lies in what it brings to our imaginations. The best lovemaking encompasses our whole bodies, not just the places where we expect to be aroused — and food contributes to the idea of sex as an all-encompassing physical experience. You could say, in other words, that it turns the whole body into an erogenous zone.

Between a 16-hour tantric session of the kind that only rock stars have the money and opportunity to indulge in and a reductive view of sex as an afterthought lies a vast landscape of sexual possibilities.

Eating together can leave us feeling cherished enough to be generous with our own affections. It reminds us that sensations of all kinds can make us

happy — and a memory of happiness can be in itself a powerful aphrodisiac.

From this awareness, it takes only a small leap of the imagination to make food part of foreplay. Experiment with the foods listed on the following pages. How do they feel — not just in your mouth, but on your skin? Avoiding hot food, think of the fun to be had in teasing your lover's expectations with different temperatures. Blindfold him or her if you wish, and don't stick to sweet goodies such as honey or ice-cream.

A delicious meal shared leaves lovers in the mood to go on spoiling each another. And if you like to precede your lovemaking with eating together, you might consider more literal-minded ways of moving from one to the next.

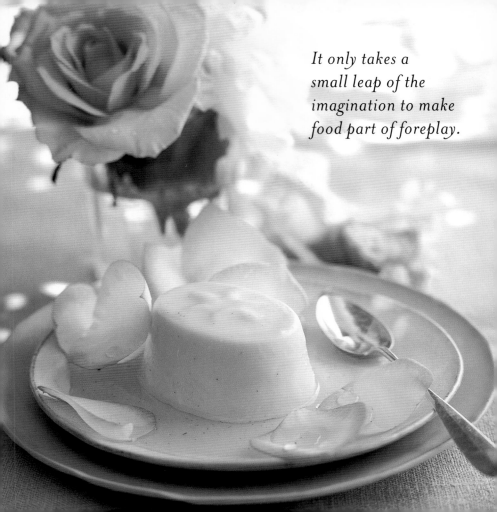

It only takes a small leap of the imagination to make food part of foreplay.

fantasy foods

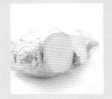

HERBS AND SPICES

Fennel and liquorice are considered to be aphrodisiacs, while various spices, especially ginger, will increase circulation in your limbs, making you feel a little pampered and bringing a flush to your cheeks.

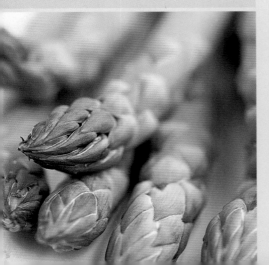

OYSTERS OR QUAILS' EGGS

Oysters are moist and velvety and slither sensually down the throat, but if they don't appeal to you, quails' eggs make a wonderful alternative starter.

ASPARAGUS

Asparagus is a phallic vegetable, and whole spears are sensual to eat. Plain-boiled and dripping with butter, English asparagus in season is unsurpassable.

FIZZ

The bubbles in champagne and sparkling wine (or even mineral water) are a great sensation to bestow on your lover's skin, especially the genital flesh, and wine is, of course, the easiest aphrodisiac to carry into the bedroom.

Asparagus is a phallic vegetable and whole spears are sensual to eat.

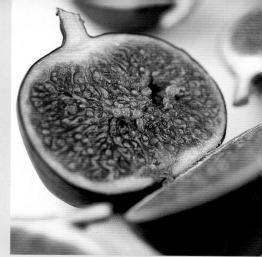

CALVES' LIVER

If you're wondering how to follow a serving of oysters, consider some calves' liver — a carnal, earthy and energy-giving treat, whether devilled or smooth and slippery like genital flesh. Serve with thin toast and a dressed rocket salad.

EXOTIC FRUITS

For a sensual and pleasantly messy treat, it's easy to create a riot of colour and texture with a plate of exotic fruits such as star fruit or fresh figs from the Mediterranean or the Middle East.

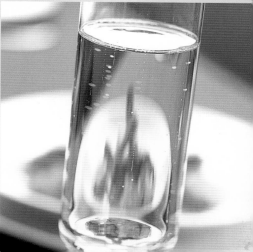

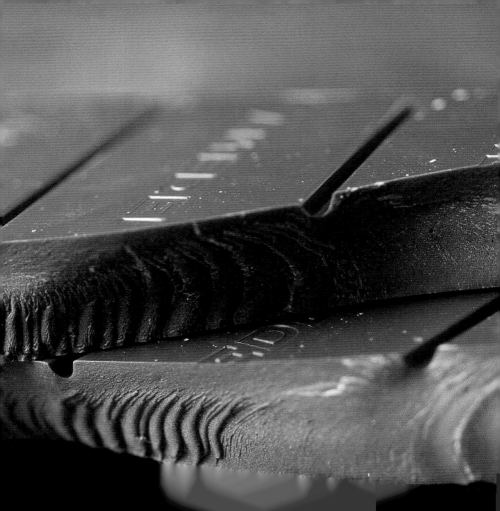

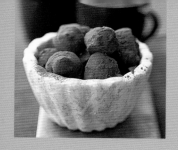

sweet delights

The chocolate residue found in a Mayan pot suggests that South Americans were drinking chocolate 2,600 years ago — the earliest recorded use of cocoa beans — while the Aztecs' lore that it was a gift from the god Quetzalcoatl suggests that they had as high an opinion of it as we do.

The great Italian lover Casanova was in no doubt about the erotic effects of drinking chocolate, describing it as 'the elixir of love', while 18th-century French doctors prescribed it for a broken heart.

Part of the sense of well-being that chocolate imparts may be the association with luxury that it has enjoyed since it arrived in Europe in the 16th century. But there is scientific evidence behind its sexy reputation too. In addition to causing the body to make the 'feel-good'

hormone serotonin, chocolate also contains phenethylamine. Produced by the harmless fermentation that occurs in chocolate after manufacture, this chemical in sufficient quantities would have the same psychotropic effects as drugs such as opium and LSD. However, phenethylamine is quickly metabolized by enzymes in the body, which prevent significant concentrations from reaching the brain, leaving us with the sense of well-being that many of us have associated with chocolate since childhood.

Solid chocolate bars, first produced in Italy and Switzerland in the 18th century, have added a lot to chocolate's aphrodisiac appeal — few things can be more suggestive than a food that melts at just below mouth temperature!

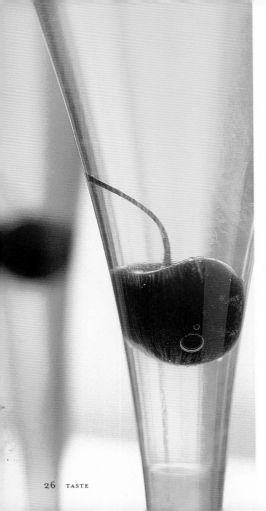

lapping it up

A small amount of alcohol relaxes you physically and emotionally. It increases your confidence, as well as making you feel flushed and warm.

Champagne is the most famously aphrodisiac wine, but three-quarters of champagne sold is non-vintage, and unless you have sampled a single-year designated vintage you can be forgiven for thinking the drink's celebratory reputation is based only on image. If you're seeking the drink's promised headiness, you won't go wrong with such a vintage, since they are produced only in the better years.

Top-notch cuvées (with quality reflected in their price, unfortunately) include Belle-Epoque from Perrier-Jouët and La Grande Dame from

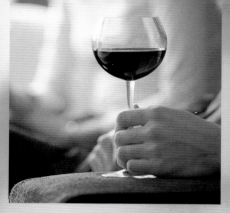
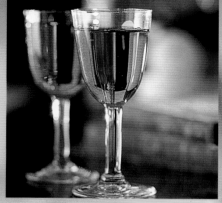

Veuve-Clicquot, while useful terms to look out for include Blanc de Blancs (made purely from chardonnay grapes) or, for a novelty, Blanc de Noirs (made only from red pinot grapes).

A decent white wine will often work just as well. Muscadet or even a bone-dry Alsace Riesling will give satisfaction as an accompaniment to oysters, fish and lightly cooked vegetables. Chardonnay has proved a hardy grape which has travelled the world. Whether French, Australian (which tend to be especially woody) or Californian, it's been the basis in recent years of an array of hugely popular wines; many are quite bland, but there are some exceptions, such as Lindemans Bin 65.

Red wines are back in vogue, but although heavy Bordeaux wines will make you feel very pampered indeed, they can also — at between 12 and 15 per cent alcohol by volume — make you sleepy and slothful, despite their sybaritic image. But Bordeaux is also the source of Sauternes, deliciously sweet, white dessert wines that have been unjustly overlooked as a seduction tool.

After such a treat, you may need some caffeine and sugar, for an energy boost.

fruits de mer

The goddess Aphrodite herself (Venus to the Romans) was said to have been borne from the sea on an oyster shell, as shown in Botticelli's painting *The Birth of Venus*, while Casanova is perhaps the most famous of Earthly oyster-lovers.

When purchasing oysters, shop so you don't drop. Go to a busy traditional fishmonger and always buy oysters live — their shells should remain closed even when tapped, and they should be quite heavy with liquor. Throw away any molluscs that are dry, shrivelled or blackish when open. It is generally advisable to eat oysters only when there's an 'R' in the name of the month — that is, at the coldest times of the year.

Native oysters (from Galway or Whitstable, for example) are preferred to Pacific, or rock, oysters, but the similarity in taste suggests that snob value plays a part in this. Rock oysters are in fact more disease-resistant and are available more often through the year.

Shucking — or opening — your oysters can be a risky business, and an oyster

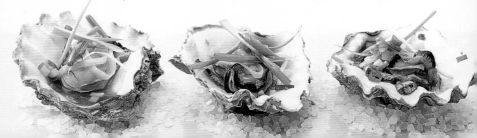

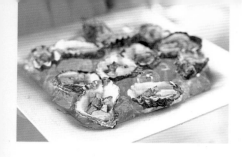

knife (with a short, round-ended blade) is a good investment if you plan to develop an oyster habit. For your safety, hold the oyster in a tea towel. Once you have wriggled off the top half of the shell, sever the tendon connecting the oyster to the shell so that it's free to slide smoothly into the mouth. Alternatively, cheat: microwave your oysters for about twenty seconds each, one at a time, or until the shell begins to open.

Oysters are cooked in a variety of ways, but the classic method of serving them raw on crushed ice (with seaweed, if you wish) remains unsurpassed when it comes to a slippery, sensual culinary experience. Lemon juice is a must, while there's no law against trying them with Worcestershire Sauce or Tabasco.

mignonette sauce

THIS SAUCE HAS A CLASSIC LIGHT TASTE THAT MAKES USE OF THE OYSTERS' OWN JUICES. THE QUANTITY PRODUCED BY THIS RECIPE IS ENOUGH TO ACCOMPANY 18 OYSTERS.

1 large glass dry white wine
1 tablespoon wine vinegar
1 shallot, finely chopped
white pepper to taste
salt (optional)

Heat the wine and vinegar in a saucepan and reduce by half. Take the pan off the heat and stir in the shallot, pepper and salt (if required — oysters tend to be salty). Add the liquor from the shucked oysters and serve the sauce separately, for your lucky 'guest' to spoon into the open half-shells.

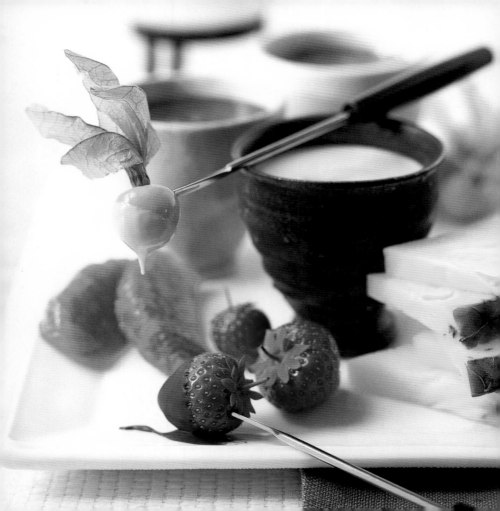

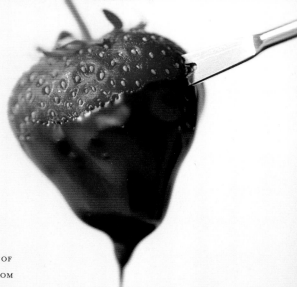

flavoursome fondue

WHEN WE FANCY SOME CHOCOLATE, MANY OF US ASSUME THAT WE MUST BE SUFFERING FROM A 'SUGAR LOW' — CRAVING SWEET THINGS IN GENERAL. BUT EVIDENCE SUGGESTS IT MAY BE THE FAMILIAR UPLIFTING EFFECTS OF THE COCOA BEAN AT WORK AS WELL. FOR A FAST, FUN AND FROLICSOME DESSERT, TAKE A TRIP BACK TO THE 1970S WITH A 'RETRO' CHOCOLATE FONDUE.

110 ml (4 fl oz) water
110 g (4 oz) sugar
400 g (14 oz) plain chocolate, broken into pieces
2 tablespoons golden syrup

Heat the water and sugar to make a syrup. Put the chocolate in a bowl and melt over a pan of simmering water. Stirring continually, add the golden syrup and enough of the sugar syrup until the mix is even and pourable. For some messy fun, serve with strawberries, grapes and citrus fruits cut into bite-sized pieces.

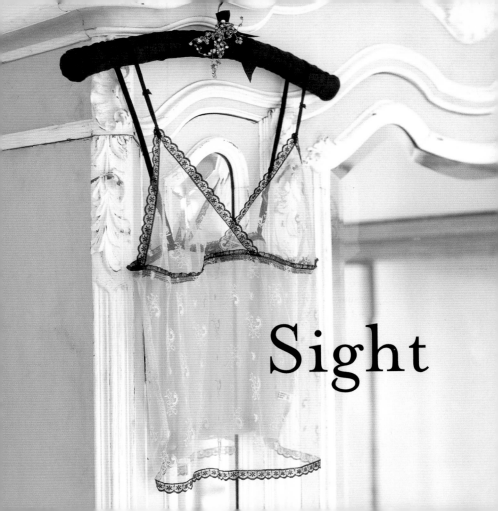

Sight

lines of beauty

Erotic visual stimuli are often associated with 'solo sex' or those occasions when we're aroused while alone, either from memory or through sights, both real and imagined, that appeal for their own sake.

We don't know why particular shapes and textures appeal to us in the way they do, but some attributes are commonly considered appealing by many people, gay and straight, male and female. We all find well-defined features attractive. In men, a tightly muscled body and bottom and a strong jaw seem to have universal sex appeal.

Make-up, meanwhile, has evolved to accentuate the natural symmetries and fine features of the female face. Women tend to be divisible into three body styles depending on the relative widths of hips and chest — the hourglass, the pear and the fuller figure — and all have their fans, together with the clothing styles that set them off best. Be confident — and don't let the fashionistas tell you what to wear in preference to a classic style that suits your particular shape. Likewise, when buying adornments such as necklaces and earrings, consider your own look and facial shape, not just the appeal of the objects themselves. Clothes in soft, muted colours accentuate the fineness of soft (or freckled) skin of any race.

Whatever your perceived physical faults, think of your appearance in a positive light and aim to accentuate what's already appealing and individual about yourself. To be at your best, be more of what you already are.

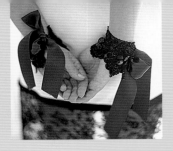

but is it art?

Poets and perverts throughout history have observed that a partially clothed body can be sexier than a naked one. Despite the association of naked flesh with free love, it seems that, when it comes to the real thing, you can't beat a bit of teasing. Leaving something to the imagination will inspire your lover to want to touch you more than anything else.

We all desire what we can't have, but it isn't just the suggestion of withholding that makes clothing attractive.

The visual hardness of straps, belts and designs that crisscross the body contrasts with the soft roundedness of flesh, delineating and framing the body and even implying a mild element of bondage. Meanwhile, sumptuous fabrics that hug the figure in all the right places, whether skimpy or long and tulip-like, are as old as the ancient world.

You may be excited by pornography or dismiss it as crude and misogynistic. If you don't fancy watching a video with your lover, consider the wide world of visual eroticism through history — of paintings and sculptures now freely displayed in galleries that were originally more at home in brothels.

From the fleshy power of Rodin's *The Kiss* to Gustav Klimt's more cruelly erotic painting of the same name, or from Reubens' rounded forms to Nobuyoshi Araki's erotic photography, artists have left us with their own sensual visions, and art books are a gentle aphrodisiac that can be left on open view for anyone to peruse.

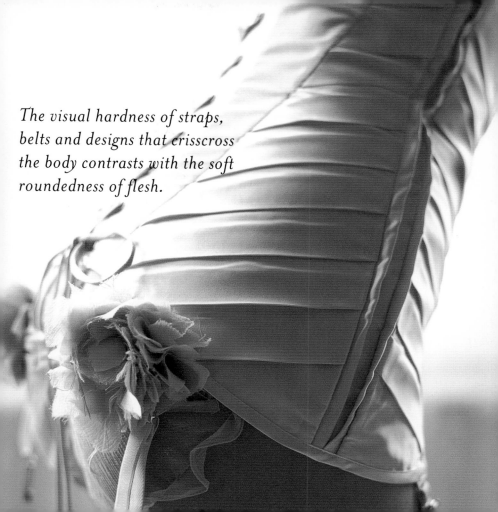

The visual hardness of straps, belts and designs that crisscross the body contrasts with the soft roundedness of flesh.

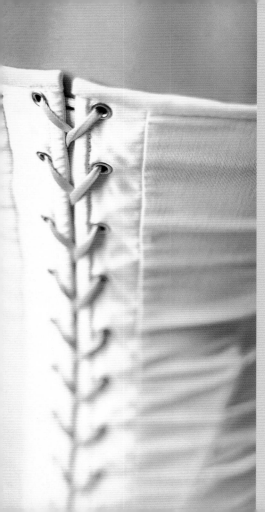

feasts for the eyes

Sight is the sense that we are culturally most aware of when it comes to being turned on. Whether with a demure wave of a fan or a flash of cheek revealed by shorts that ride high, different societies all have their accepted ways of showing what's on our minds. But each of us, too, has our private, intimate visual turn-ons. What are yours? They could be any — or none — in the list opposite.

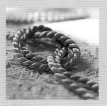

Seductive signals take a myriad different forms.

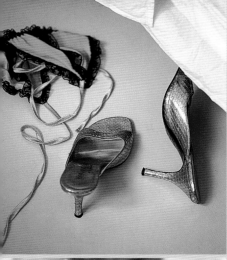

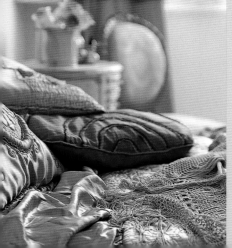

The way your lover shakes her hair
or takes off his glasses.

✳

The sight of a place — a bedroom, a car,
a cornfield — you would like, or are going,
to make love in.

✳

Whether shopping for your partner,
or just looking, the clothes — in stores
or on others — that you'd like to
see your partner wearing.

✳

People in uniform.

✳

Your lover's eyes, when you know what
he or she is thinking.

✳

The sight of innocent objects that you could use
as part of a kinky sex-game with your lover,
or maybe have already used in such a way.

✳

Boxers or briefs? Lacy Bravissimo,
colourful Agent Provocateur or a bespoke
waspy corset from Rigby & Peller?

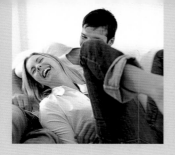

the language of desire

Whether or not we are aware of it, we all use body language. The visual messages we send out are interpreted as indicating our desires as much as the words that come out of our mouths. Aphrodisiac gestures and behaviour can help our seduction along at an almost unconscious level, until we are ready to make our eagerness screamingly obvious.

HAIR PLAY

Long hair gives more scope for seductive glances; playing with your hair indicates that you'd like to be played with yourself.

FULL-ON FEET

People tend to point their feet towards a person they're interested in, facing that person full-on. Touch your legs, and your partner's likely to contemplate doing the same. In fact, the more interested we are, the more we tend to copy someone's body language altogether.

LIP LICKING

Our lips become swollen and red when we are aroused. Lipstick (and even collagen) evolved to mimic this. Lovers can't help focusing on each other's lips; if you are the subject of such interest, reward your partner by licking and moistening your lips a little.

HANGING LOOSE

Holding your arms to your sides sends out an offputting message, while showing your palms and the undersides of your forearms is inviting.

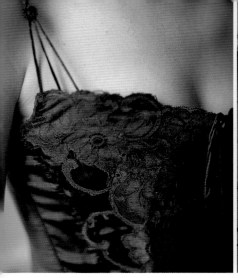

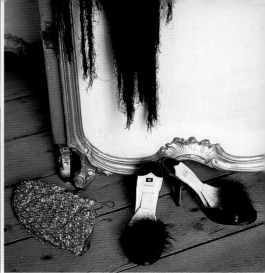

A MATTER OF SHAPE

Shoulders are an area in which gender differences are visible. While women find broad shoulders attractive in men, women's bare shoulders, smooth and round, can seem especially feminine.

EYEING UP

The pupils of our eyes widen when we feel sexually interest in someone and also — conveniently — in low light.

Our lips are swollen and red when we are aroused.

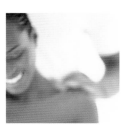

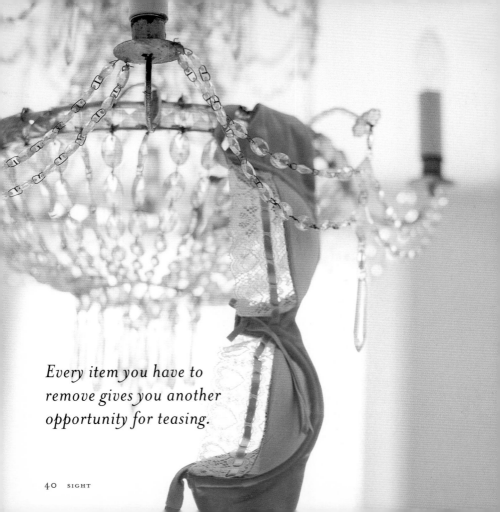

*Every item you have to
remove gives you another
opportunity for teasing.*

teaserama

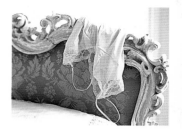

Recent surveys have shown that stripping seductively for an audience of one — or more — is the prime female fantasy. So it is far from unusual to enjoy the idea of showing off for your lover.

There are a few simple steps that can help to make the reality of striptease just as enjoyable. A fantasist can invent the environment in which a fantasy takes place. When it comes to reality, try to be as in control of your surroundings as possible, and make them work for you.

Location is everything — it would be more than a little poignant if you came on like a burlesque babe in front of a tatty old broom cupboard!

As discussed in Touch, you should take account of how you are lit. Avoid harsh light, which flattens, rather than flatters, features and curves. Make sure your light sources are low, or dimmable, and draw the curtains. Meanwhile, think about the creatively raunchy use you can make of fixtures, fittings and furniture — all in the name of art, of course.

Consider the ways in which you can frame your body by means of underwear, footwear, neckwear and hair. Put on your clothes in the reverse order to the one in which you'll undress, especially when it comes to suspender belts and knickers — and wear as much as you want. Every item you have to remove gives you another opportunity for teasing.

Be true to yourself: if you generally feel more proper than a pole-dancer, assume that attitude and remove it piece by piece. Let your hair down — literally.

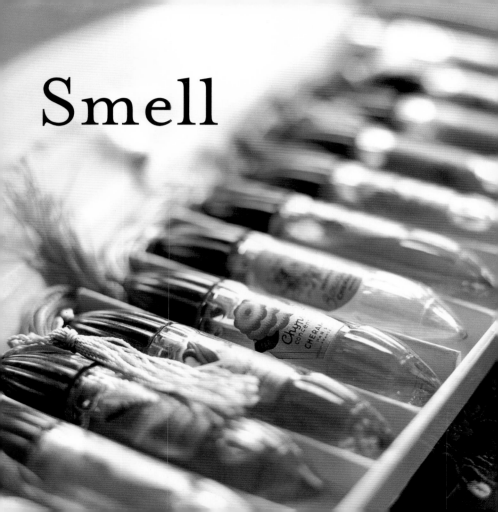

Smell

animal
instincts

Smell is the most deeply affecting of all our senses. It is the sense of which we are usually the least conscious unless we have cause to recognize especially pleasant, unpleasant or alarming scents. We are inclined to think of smells in terms of particular uses, for their purely practical value. They allow us to check whether, for example, food is fresh, a baby needs changing, or a fire is burning.

We underestimate the importance of our sense of smell — perhaps because to lose it would not alter the way we live our lives as radically as the loss of sight or hearing. Yet our sense of smell intertwines uniquely with our memories to affect mood and happiness. Years after an event, the odour of its time and place can make us wistful or inexplicably

happy, without our necessarily being conscious that the scents around us may be contributing to our mood, let alone why. This may be particularly true when it comes to aphrodisiac smells.

The existence and purpose of human pheromones — chemicals that relay a fact about an animal, such as its level of fertility, to other members of the same species — have become subjects of hot debate thanks to their exploitation by unscrupulous hucksters.

But, since the 1990s, scientists have found evidence that hormonal changes can occur in a human being in response to another person's body odour alone, and that we respond to others' scents, even in isolation, according to our sexual orientation.

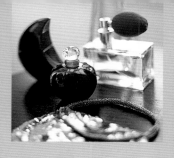

capturing the right notes

It is a short step from acknowledging the psychological importance of smell to manipulating it. Most of us practise some form of aromatherapy — walking through a sweet-smelling garden, burning a scented candle — without thinking of it in those terms. In fact, not only our perfumes but many of our mass-market beauty products are based on aromatherapy techniques.

There is no scientific explanation for the effects of aromatherapy. Although many essential oils have an antimicrobial use, this is separate from the role they play in aromatherapy, in which the smell alone is said to heal, uplift and arouse.

Essential oils are concentrated from aromatic plants and can be expensive due to the large number of plants required to make them, but only a few drops of oil at a time are needed to achieve the desired effect.

Rather like wines, essential oils are rated in terms of 'notes' — top notes, middle notes and base notes — which vary according to their rate of evaporation and therefore how long their scent lasts.

There are no fixed rules about how to blend your oils, but a combination of all three notes will work best. With a little experimentation, you'll find a blend that's right for you (see pages 49–51).

TOP NOTES are the most uplifting. Strongly scented, they last for between three and 24 hours. Good examples are basil, bergamot, eucalyptus, neroli, peppermint and thyme.

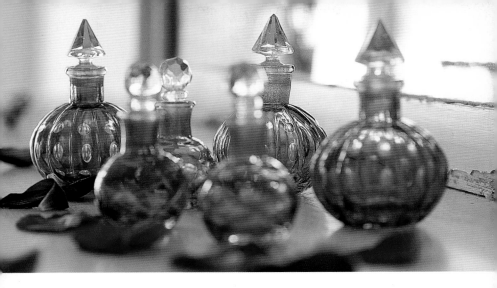

MIDDLE NOTES come next, lasting two to three days, and are less perfumed than top-note oils. Examples include chamomile, fennel, juniper, lavender and rosemary.

BASE NOTES, being the slowest to evaporate, can last for up to a week. They are generally soothing and relaxing. Examples include cedar, clove, ginger, jasmine and sandalwood.

The smell alone is said to heal, uplift and arouse.

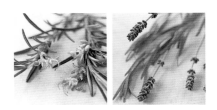

perfumes & passion

Perfume manufacturers have made fortunes creating artificial fragrances that promise to make us irresistible to our lovers or potential lovers, but most of the smells that can turn us on — or remind us of the good times — are to be found in nature.

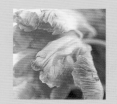

THE WONDERFUL SCENTS OF SPRING
Sir John Harington, a courtier during the reign of Queen Elizabeth I, wrote, 'A young man and a young woman in a green arbor on a May morning — if God do not forgive it, I would.'

... OR SUMMER
The smell of sun-tan oil or lotion — a practical necessity that can be part of an erotic grooming ritual too.

... OR WINTER
The aroma of a real coal fire, best experienced from a cosy hearth rug!

FLOWERS AND PLANTS
The fragrance of rose or orange blossom — which, like neroli, is a seductive staple of aromatherapy.

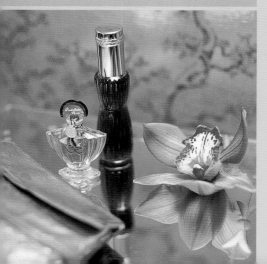

TREES
Pine, cedar and other scents associated with a romantic woodland stroll.

A LOVER'S BREATH
The smell of your lover's fresh breath, hot on your cheek, as you begin to kiss.

BODY ODOURS
We laugh at them — but we all have our very own, and they play a crucial role in sexual arousal. Who hasn't sniffed the clothes of a much-missed lover?

GORGEOUS FOOD AROMAS
They can bring back memories of sexually charged evenings. Italian foods are a favourite, especially those that include fresh herbs such as basil.

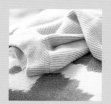

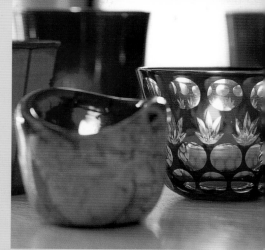

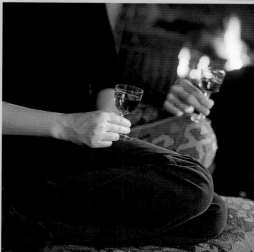

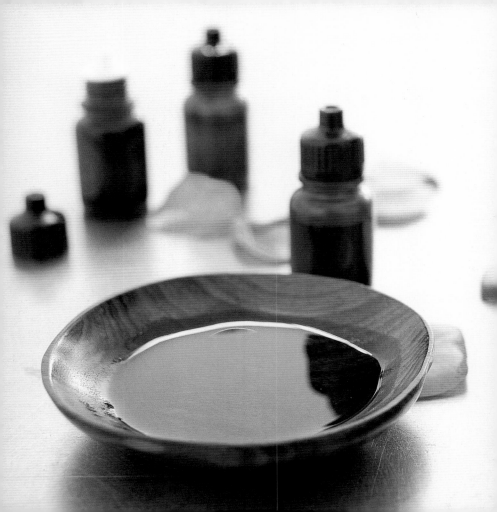

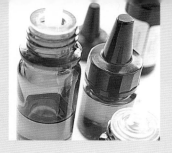

oiling the works

Whether you want to feel totally relaxed or deliciously tantalized, aromatherapy can add an entirely new dimension to a massage (see pages 16–17) and is a marvellous way to maximize its effects. During an aromatherapy massage, essential oils are absorbed through the skin as well as being inhaled.

Essential oils cause irritation when applied directly to the skin, so always dilute them in a carrier oil. Popular carrier oils include almond, which is easily absorbed and contains vitamin D; avocado, an effective emollient for dry skin; hazelnut, a sensuous, light oil rich in vitamin E; and peach kernel oil, which contains vitamins A and E.

Some essential oils can take up to two hours to absorb, so, to achieve the most potent effect, don't let your subject shower too soon after the massage.

Using a stoppered container, blend 15 drops of your chosen essential oils with 250 ml (1 fl oz) of a carrier oil and shake very well. (Once blended, oils turn rancid quite fast, so if you make too much of a mixture, store it in a cool, dark place and it may last up to three months.)

Popular essential oils for massage, whether applied to the skin or vaporized to enhance the atmosphere around you include the following: basil, bergamot, orange, clary sage, eucalyptus, jasmine, lavender, sandalwood, rose — a great aphrodisiac scent — and ylang ylang from the cananga tree. In Indonesia, ylang ylang leaves are traditionally spread on the marital bed of newlyweds.

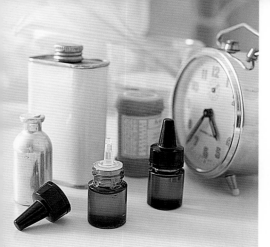

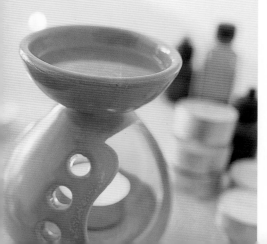

seductive combinations

The key to developing your own oils is to determine what it is you want to use them for. This section focuses on fresh combinations that will relax, pamper and seduce, but be aware that the real appeal of aromatherapy lies in being able to concoct your own blends.

FOR A SWEATILY SEXY BUT HEALING MASSAGE OIL

3 drops clary sage
4 drops eucalyptus
115 ml carrier oil such as almond or avocado

FOR A LESS PUNGENT ALTERNATIVE

4 drops lavender
4 drops eucalyptus
130 ml carrier oil such as almond or avocado

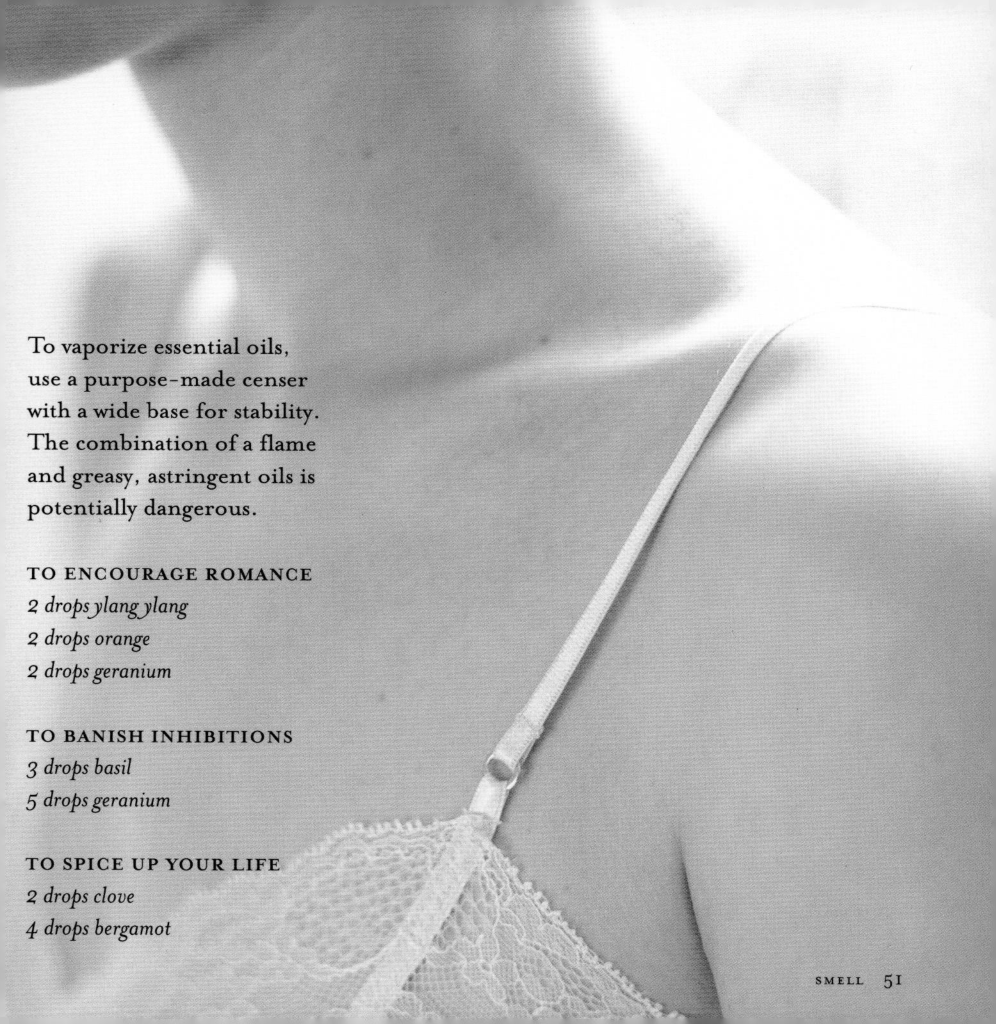

To vaporize essential oils,
use a purpose-made censer
with a wide base for stability.
The combination of a flame
and greasy, astringent oils is
potentially dangerous.

TO ENCOURAGE ROMANCE
2 drops ylang ylang
2 drops orange
2 drops geranium

TO BANISH INHIBITIONS
3 drops basil
5 drops geranium

TO SPICE UP YOUR LIFE
2 drops clove
4 drops bergamot

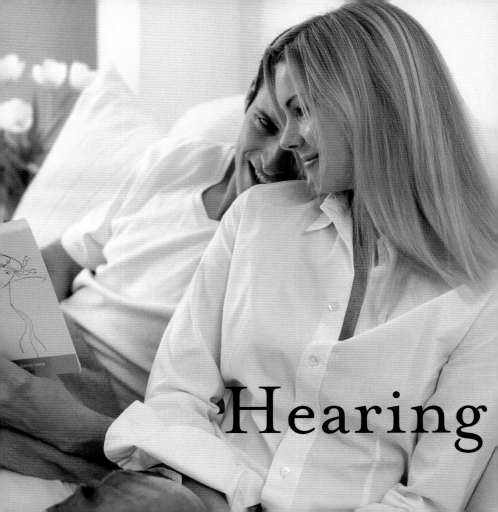

Hearing

the sounds of sex

It is easy to overlook the influence of sounds on sexual arousal. When we are absent from our partner, we are inclined to recall love and lovemaking in terms of images. But, when the time is right, all kinds of sounds contribute to our arousal, whether or not we are aware of them having this effect – and not just the moans and grunts that first come to mind. Each of us, if we think about it, has a few pet sounds – particular noises whose waves caress our ears like the tip of a lover's tongue.

The sound that turns you on most powerfully could be the quality of your partner's voice itself, its confidence or vulnerability; its depth or lightness of tone. More raunchily, you could be stimulated by the wet sound of a kiss; the rustlings and unbucklings of clothes coming off in a hurry; even the rhythmic swishing of a crop or a cane.

This is not to ignore the many different sounds involved in lovemaking itself. Maybe the rustle of a condom wrapper makes you prick up your ears like Pavlov's dog – or the stimulus could be as simple as the sense of well-being created by the popping of a cork and the clink of glasses.

Whatever sounds boost your state of arousal, make your partner aware of them. Become aware of yourself and of your lover and tune into your own personal soundtrack at any stage of sex or seduction.

de-lightful

The American singer James Brown put the case succinctly when he told us that he would 'stay on the scene like a sex machine'. Throughout recorded history, music has put humankind in the mood for licentious revels and provided a soundtrack for sexual frolics. It has also captured the most wistful, soulful and longing sentiments for others that it is possible to feel.

Listen to what your lover likes. Some of us enjoy sharing our tastes with others and like to assume we know best, but we all have something to give, and in being open to other people's tastes we often find the route to wonderful areas of music that we may not have encountered before. Music generally represents the best and most sensitive aspects of any culture — as well as, sometimes, its darker sides — which is why it has always been considered an ambassador for love, let alone for world peace.

Classical music can be sexier and sleazier than buttoned-up images of symphony orchestras suggest, while many tracks reflect how mellow and reflective pop music can be.

Consider, for example, how the grandness of opera obscures the fact that most of its storylines are lust-filled dramas full of the dizzy heights and deep lows of obsessive love, whose characters live or die by their passions — in low-life settings such as brothels and bars as often as in palaces and parliaments.

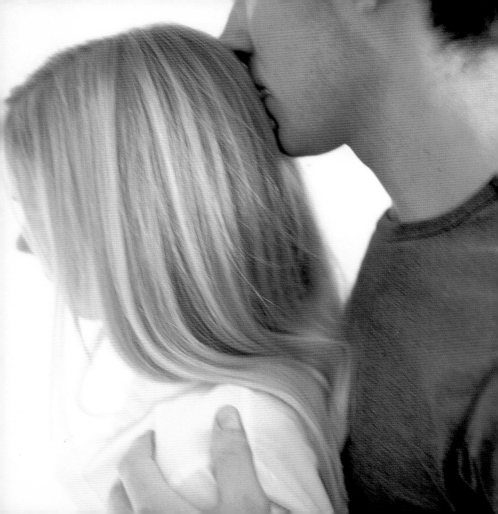

love for sale

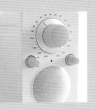

No one can tell anyone else what to like — and the sound of cheap, squeaky bedsprings may be what does it for you — but the following list of musical temptations may include at least some items that could intensify the sensual quality of your love life.

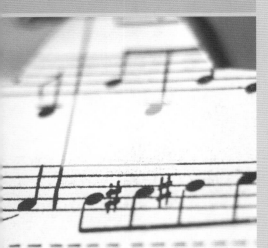

A sense of good living is a strong turn-on in itself.

The 1990s revived the popularity of Gregorian chant through chilled-out music by bands such as Enigma. Less clichéd and even more relaxing are the female voices of early oratorios by Hildegard von Bingen (1098–1179).

Likewise, we are all familiar with guitar heroes — and they go back a long way. John Dowland (1563–1626) was an Elizabethan 'lute hero' who produced some of the most romantic and tender tunes ever.

Opera is a feast for the senses. A sense of good living has an aphrodisiac value in itself. Sexily listenable examples of classical music include:

Mozart's *Don Giovanni* (1787)

✳

Donizetti's *Lucia de Lammermoor* (1835)

✳

Britten's *Young Person's Guide to the Orchestra*
(1946)

✳

Alban Berg's *Lulu* (1947)

Less misogynistic than the casino
crooners of the Rat Pack, these torch
singers will make any listener feel as
seductive as a sophisticated Manhattanite.
Check out the songs of:

Jerome Kern
George and Ira Gershwin
Cole Porter

…as sung by the likes of:

Ella Fitzgerald
Billie Holiday
Bessie Smith
Nina Simone

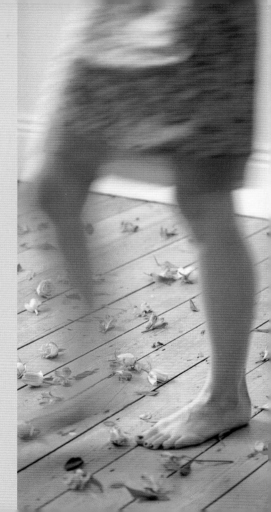

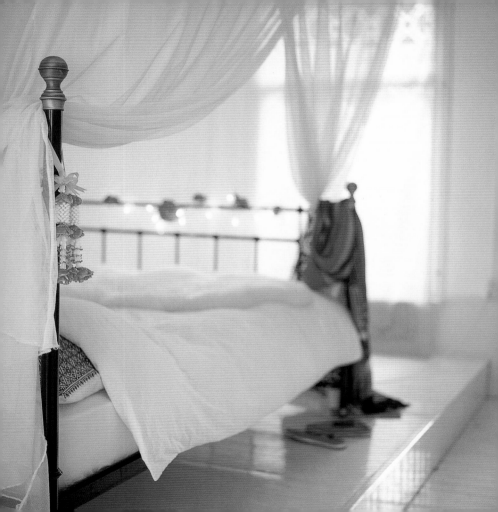

de-lovely

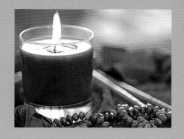

From the earliest civilizations people are known to have danced and flaunted themselves for seductive purposes on ritual occasions. Today, we have pop stars to do it for us. Elvis, Madonna, Mick, Robbie, Britney, Christina and company give us an image of their sexual selves to reflect aspects of our own, to a backbeat that inspires us to move our hips the way we do when we make love.

But when it comes to the act of sexual intercourse itself, lyrics can get in the way. Thankfully, the spirit of 1990s European dance music has been married to mellow ambient sounds to produce a lush aural cocktail that is perfect for the bedroom, and practised by the likes of Air and Goldfrapp.

Meanwhile, erotic dance styles from burlesque to belly dancing are back in vogue, so if you are feeling playful enough to gyrate or strip for your partner (see pages 40–41), you are free to draw your inspiration from *New York, New York* rather than *Total Eclipse of the Heart*.

As for the ups and downs of oral culture, the spoken word has more than a small part to play not just in discussing love and lovemaking but in turning us on, too. Some of us may be fortunate enough to have a partner who has the confidence, and talent for timing, to share their fantasies with us during sex — the verbal and mental equivalent of a striptease — or even narrate our own fantasies back to us.

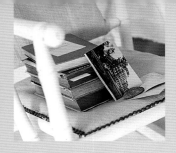

sweet nothings

If you are feeling slightly short of sexual inspiration, remember that not all erotic literature is produced for a dirty-mac brigade, nor is all romantic fiction bland. Leaving aside the intellectualism of fetish writers such as the Marquis de Sade or Mirbeau, and the plain heavy-going of D. H. Lawrence's *Lady Chatterley's Lover*, there is a treasure-trove of writings by those who have sought to arouse. From bohemians Anaïs Nin and Henry Miller to eroticists such as Marguerite Duras or Alina Reyes and modern writers such as Nicholson Baker, there is a wealth of material beside the mainstream 'bonkbusters' that give us guilty pleasure.

Oscar Wilde famously quipped that the best drug known to humankind is good conversation. Try reading aloud to your partner — it's a treat that can make the hardest of us feel like a pampered child. It can open new pathways of communication and introduce aspects of sex you haven't shared before. (And it isn't a bad way to do that, if that's what you want to achieve.)

In Shakespeare's *The Merry Wives of Windsor*, Falstaff calls for a rain of exotic Elizabethan aphrodisiacs to fall from the sky. But Falstaff is a comic character mainly because he is inspired not by love but money, whereas the most arousing turn-on of all — our eagerness for our partner — can't be faked. From talking dirty to romantic longing, it really is the thought that counts.

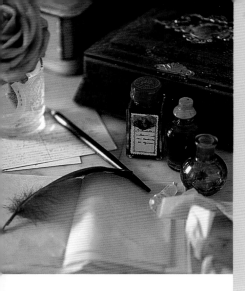

Wild nights! Wild nights!
Were I with thee,
Wild nights should be
Our luxury!

Futile the winds
To a heart in port, —
Done with the compass,
Done with the chart.

Rowing in Eden!
Ah! The sea!
Might I but moor
To-night in thee!

WILD NIGHTS
BY EMILY DICKINSON (1830–86)

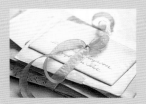

Your hand in my hand,
My soul inspired
My heart in bliss,
Because we go together.

ANCIENT EGYPTIAN LOVE POEM,
2000–1100 BC

index